# Oral Sex Handbook for Couples in Love

## A Complete Guide to Oral Sex and Tips to Make It More Enjoyable for Romantic Couples

Cheryl Bach

# Oral Sex Handbook for Couples in Love

©2024 by Cheryl Bach



Publisher: IntimateInk Press

Email: intimateinkpress@gmail.com

This book is a work of nonfiction intended for informational purposes only. The content of this book is based on the author's research, knowledge, and experience, and it is provided with the understanding that the author and publisher are not engaged in rendering legal, medical, or professional advice. The information in this book is not a substitute for professional guidance or assistance. Readers should consult with relevant professionals for advice and assistance regarding their specific situations. The author and publisher disclaim any liability for any loss or risk, personal or otherwise, which is incurred as a consequence, directly or indirectly, of the use and application of any of the contents of this book.

Cover design by IntimateInk Press

Interior layout and design by IntimateInk Press

Printed in USA

Fonts: Google fonts

Image: Freepik.com. This cover has been designed using assets from Freepik.com

For permission to use copyrighted material from this book, please contact the copyright holder listed above.

First Edition: 2024

Distributed by Amazon.com, Inc.

# Table of Contents

# **Introduction**

Welcome to "Oral Sex Handbook for Couples in Love: A Complete Guide to Oral Sex and Tips to Make It More Enjoyable for Romantic Couples". From the first kiss to the most intimate of moments, oral sex is an important element of a fulfilling sex life. However, it can be both confusing and daunting, especially for couples new to exploring this practice.

This book will provide you with a comprehensive guide to oral sex, packed with tips and ideas for making it a more enjoyable and satisfying experience for both partners. We will dive into the anatomy, techniques, and positions that can help you achieve heightened pleasure, as well as explore common concerns and questions couples may have.

Oral Sex Handbook for Couples in Love

As we journey through the various aspects of oral sex, we will emphasize the importance of communication, consent, and trust. Communication is key to ensuring that both partners are comfortable and feeling their best. Consent is essential to any sexual experience, and trust is crucial to building intimacy and pleasure in a relationship.

Throughout this book, we will also encourage couples to experiment with new ideas and techniques, tailored to their unique preferences and desires. Whether you're looking to spice up your foreplay routine or take things to the next level, there is something for every couple in this guide.

In addition to exploring techniques and positions, we will also discuss strategies for overcoming common challenges like gag reflex, dental dams, and hygiene concerns. We will also explore important tips for giving and receiving oral sex, including tricks for stamina, finding the right rhythm, and creating an atmosphere of intimacy and excitement.

Cheryl Bach

We believe that oral sex should be a fun and fulfilling part of any couple's sex life. With this handbook, we hope to provide you with the tools and knowledge to make oral sex a joyful and intimate part of your relationship.

We invite you to open yourself up to the world of oral sex, to explore a new level of intimacy with your partner, and to discover the pleasures that come from putting your trust in each other. So, let's dive in and get started on this exciting journey!

# Chapter 1

## Understanding Oral Sex

Whether you're brand new to oral sex or a seasoned pro, it's essential to understand the basics. In this chapter, we'll dive into what it is, the benefits for both the giver and receiver, and clear up some common misconceptions.

**What Is Oral Sex?**

Oral sex, also known as cunnilingus or fellatio, is when one partner engages in sexual pleasure with the mouth, tongue, and lips of the other partner's genital area. It can be a part of foreplay or the main event, depending on your preferences as a couple.

**Benefits of Oral Sex**

The benefits of oral sex are numerous, and they apply to both the giver and receiver. For the receiver, oral sex can offer intense pleasure and can be a way to achieve orgasm without penetration. For the giver, providing oral sex can be a way to connect with their partner on a deeper level and can be a turn-on for many people. Additionally, oral sex is a form of safe sex, which can reduce the risk of sexually transmitted infections or unwanted pregnancy.

**Clearing Up Common Misconceptions**

As with any sexual act, there are many misconceptions about oral sex. One common misconception is that it is only for young people or those in casual relationships, but this is simply not true. Oral sex can be a part of any healthy sexual relationship, regardless of age or relationship status.

Another misconception is that oral sex is dirty or shameful. This belief is rooted in societal taboos surrounding sexuality, particularly female sexuality. However, oral sex can be a beautiful expression of intimacy and pleasure between two consenting adults.

It's also important to understand that everyone's preferences and limits are different. Some people may love receiving oral sex and may find it incredibly pleasurable, while others may not enjoy it as much. Similarly, some people may enjoy giving oral sex, while others may not feel comfortable with it. It's important to communicate with your partner and respect each other's boundaries and preferences.

In conclusion, understanding the basics of oral sex is crucial for building a fulfilling and mutually satisfying sexual relationship with your partner. By exploring the benefits for both the giver and receiver and clearing up common misconceptions, you can broaden your perspectives and deepen your connection with your partner.

Remember, like any sexual activity, communication, consent, and mutual respect are key to a positive experience. Take time to discuss your desires, boundaries, and expectations with your partner and always prioritize each other's comfort and pleasure. In the next chapter, we'll explore some tips and techniques for enhancing your oral sex experiences.

# Chapter 2

## Prepping for the Main Event

Oral sex is a sensual experience that requires some preparation, both physically and emotionally. Since every person is different, it's important to engage in open communication with your partner about your likes and dislikes to ensure a pleasurable experience. This chapter will discuss basic hygiene and grooming tips, as well as how you can create a comfortable and intimate environment for oral sex.

**Basic Hygiene and Grooming Tips**

Before engaging in oral sex, it's important to be mindful of basic hygiene practices. Make sure to take a shower or bath before indulging in oral sex, as this helps eliminate bacteria that may cause infections. Pay extra attention to your genital area, using mild soap to clean and rinse thoroughly.

Trimming or shaving your pubic hair is a personal preference, but many find it makes for a cleaner and smoother experience. However, it's important to avoid shaving right before engaging in oral sex, as this can cause irritation or razor burn to your partner's sensitive areas.

Ensure that your breath is fresh by brushing your teeth and tongue thoroughly and using mouthwash. Avoid consuming foods with strong flavors or odors before engaging in oral sex to prevent unpleasant tastes or smells.

**Creating a Comfortable, Intimate Environment**

Oral sex is an intimate experience that requires a comfortable environment. Start by selecting a private and quiet location where you won't be interrupted by anyone.

Ensure that the room's temperature is warm enough to prevent any discomfort.

Create a romantic ambiance by dimming the lights, playing soft music, and lighting candles.

You can also decorate the room with some fresh flowers or other decorative pieces that fit the mood. Setting the mood in this way helps in creating a relaxed atmosphere and can enhance arousal.

Take care of your partner's comfort by providing some pillows or cushions to support them in a comfortable position. If you have pets, it's better to keep them out of the room to avoid any distractions.

# Chapter 3

## Getting Started

Oral sex can be an incredibly intimate and pleasurable experience for couples in love. Communicating with your partner about what you both enjoy is essential to set the stage for a comfortable and enjoyable experience. Building anticipation and setting the mood can enhance arousal and create an atmosphere of complete intimacy.

**Communication with Your Partner**

Communication with your partner is the key to successful oral sex. Oral sex can be a very personal experience, and what feels good to one person may not feel pleasant to another. It's important to have open, candid conversations with your partner before engaging in any sexual activity, especially oral sex. These conversations help build trust and establish boundaries that lead to a more enjoyable and satisfying experience.

Before engaging in oral sex, sit down with your partner in an atmosphere that's conducive to personal communication, such as a quiet room where you won't be heard. Start by discussing your feelings and any concerns or hesitations you may have. It's essential to create a non-judgmental, safe space where both partners can express their desires and share any reservations or vulnerabilities that could affect their pleasure.

As you continue the conversation, express what you enjoy and what you don't enjoy when it comes to oral sex. Make sure to listen carefully to what your partner is saying so that you can understand their needs and boundaries. It's important to be honest and respectful in your communication to ensure that both partners feel comfortable and confident.

## Building Anticipation and Setting the Mood

Building anticipation is an essential part of making oral sex more enjoyable. The more aroused both partners are, the more pleasurable the experience will be. Setting the mood and creating a relaxed environment can help increase arousal and create an atmosphere that's romantic, intimate, and sensual. Here are some tips to help you get started:

**Create a Romantic Atmosphere**: Consider lighting candles or dimming the lights to create a romantic atmosphere that promotes relaxation and intimacy. Soft music, fresh flowers, or scented oils can also enhance the ambiance and help you and your partner relax.

**Use Sexual Tension**: Sexual tension builds anticipation and adds spice to a sexual encounter. You can use flirting, teasing, or even suggestive eye contact to help build this tension before engaging in oral sex.

**Take Things Slow**: Moving slowly and sensually can prolong the pleasure and create a more intimate experience. Take your time kissing, caressing, and exploring each other's bodies before diving into the main event. This will help you and your partner feel more relaxed and more connected.

**Focus on Foreplay:** Foreplay is crucial to oral sex. Start by touching and kissing your partner's body all over, including their erogenous zones. This will help build up tension and anticipation, making the experience more enjoyable for both of you. You can also consider using your hands or other toys during foreplay to help increase arousal.

**Respect Boundaries**: It's important to respect each other's boundaries before, during, and after oral sex. This includes getting consent from your partner before engaging in any sexual activity and stopping if either partner feels uncomfortable or needs a break. This will help create an atmosphere of mutual trust and respect.

**Pay Attention to Hygiene**: Good hygiene is essential for an enjoyable oral sex experience. Make sure to clean yourself thoroughly before engaging in any sexual activity. You can also consider showering together beforehand, which can enhance intimacy and create a clean and fresh environment.

**Mix it Up**: Variation is the spice of life, and this applies to oral sex too. Trying out different positions, techniques, and rhythms can help keep things interesting and prevent the experience from becoming monotonous. Pay attention to your partner's reactions and adjust your approach accordingly.

In conclusion, communication and setting the mood are crucial to having a pleasurable and memorable experience with your partner. Building anticipation, taking things slow, and paying attention to hygiene can also make a big difference. Remember to prioritize your partner's comfort and to respect each other's boundaries at all times. With these tips in mind, you can look forward to enjoying oral sex as a couple in love.

# Chapter 4

## Techniques and Tips for Beginners

Oral sex is an incredibly intimate experience that can bring pleasure to you and your partner. For beginners, it might seem confusing or intimidating to give and receive oral sex. But don't worry; with patience, practice, and communication, you'll learn how to make oral sex a pleasurable experience for both you and your partner. In this chapter, we will explore some basic techniques and tips for beginners and highlight some common mistakes to avoid while engaging in oral sex.

## Techniques for Beginners

Oral sex techniques vary from person to person, but there are some basic guidelines that can help beginners improve their skill and intimacy.

**Here are some techniques you could try:**

**The Lick-and-Suck Technique**: Begin by licking the area around your partner's vulva or penis with your tongue. Try using flat, wide strokes or flicks of your tongue. Increase pressure as desired by using the tip of your tongue and gently suck on the genital area.

**The "O" Technique**: Shaping your lips into an "O" and positioning them around your partner's clitoris or penis can create a gentle suction and stimulate blood flow. Use your tongue to flick back and forth, either side to side or up and down, and incorporate different rhythms to build arousal.

**The Use of Teeth**: Using teeth can enhance pleasure but it is critical to be cautious. Ideally, use teeth only when your partner prefers it and start gentle. Start by nibbling and using teeth around the edges of the genital area with caution.

**The Combination Technique:** Combining various techniques for more pleasurable and varied experiences. For instance, you could try alternating between using your tongue and fingers, or using different tongue movements like circling or flicking while softly sucking or using your lips in different shapes.

**Communication**: Keep the line of communication open with your partner throughout. Ask their preferences and adjust your techniques accordingly to make the experience more enjoyable for both of you.

**Common Mistakes to Avoid**

Although there are many ways to make oral sex an amazing experience, it is important to avoid some common mistakes that could be unpleasant or even painful for your partner.

**Here are a few tips to help you avoid those mistakes:**

Skipping foreplay and rushing into oral sex can often be a mistake. Foreplay helps build intimacy and excitement, and it's crucial for both partners to achieve maximum pleasure.

Neglecting hygiene is another common mistake. Before engaging in oral sex, make sure you and your partner are clean and odor-free. Oral sex can be unpleasant if either partner is not clean.

Using teeth too aggressively can cause pain and discomfort for your partner. Use your teeth with caution, and always start slow, gentle and ask your partner their preference about using teeth during oral sex.

Be aware of your partner's comfort level and don't neglect non-verbal communication. Pay attention to your partner's reactions, their breathing, and how they respond to the techniques you use. If at any point your partner seems uncomfortable or needs a break, it's important to respect that and slow down or stop.

In conclusion, with patience, practice, and communication, oral sex can be a mutually enjoyable and intimate experience for partners in a romantic relationship. Experimenting with different techniques and avoiding common mistakes can help beginners to navigate this sexual terrain with ease.

Remember, consent is key, avoid mistakes by communicating with your partner, keep hygiene in check, be mindful of your partner's comfort level, and don't forget to have fun and enjoy the experience together. Oral sex can be incredibly rewarding for both partners if done well, so take your time, relax, and explore different techniques that suit you and your partner's mutual preferences.

Cheryl Bach

# Chapter 5

## Advanced Techniques for Pros

If you've been giving and receiving oral sex for some time now, you might be looking to take your skills to the next level. This chapter provides you with tips and techniques to try out with your partner that can add new dimensions of pleasure to your intimate experiences.

**Techniques for Experienced Givers**

As an experienced giver, you already have a good handle on how to use your mouth and tongue on your partner. However, there are a few advanced techniques you can try to freshen things up and take your skills to the next level.

Cheryl Bach

One technique you can try is using your hands in addition to your mouth. While using your mouth on the head of your partner's penis, try stroking the underside of their shaft with one hand. Alternatively, you could use two hands to provide more control and sensation at the same time.

Another advanced technique that you can try out is the use of deep-throating. Deep throating involves taking your partner's entire penis into your mouth and down your throat. It requires some practice and preparation, but it can add a whole new level of pleasure to your oral sex sessions. A good trick for practicing deep-throating is to try to relax your throat muscles, which will help you ease the penis further back in your mouth.

If your partner enjoys anal play, you can also incorporate this into your oral sex routine. Using your tongue, you can stimulate your partner's perineum, the area between the scrotum and the anus. You can even gently insert your tongue into their anus if they are comfortable with it.

## How to Take Your Skills to the Next Level

One effective way to take your oral sex skills to the next level is by being fully present and attentive during the experience. To do this, try focusing on different parts of your partner's body. Pay attention to their breathing, the way their muscles tense and relax, and any sounds they make. By tuning in to your partner's reactions, you'll be able to better gauge what techniques they're enjoying and what areas are more sensitive than others.

Another way to enhance the experience is to communicate openly with your partner. Ask them what they enjoy and what they want more of. You can also experiment with new positions or techniques together, making sure to check in with each other along the way.

Lastly, incorporating toys such as vibrators or masturbators into your routine can add a whole new dimension of pleasure for you both. These toys can be used in combination with oral sex, or on their own to switch things up.

In conclusion, by incorporating a combination of different techniques, being fully present, communicating openly with your partner, and experimenting with new ideas and toys, you can take your oral sex skills to the next level. Remember to always prioritize your partner's pleasure and comfort, and never be afraid to try new things and have fun together.

# Chapter 6

## Mixing It Up

In any relationship, keeping things new and exciting in the bedroom is essential for maintaining satisfaction and fulfillment. This chapter will guide you through some creative ideas to mix things up in your oral sex routine, keeping it enjoyable and fun.

**Ideas for Creative and Exciting Experiences**

One way to mix things up is to try out different positions or locations. Oral sex doesn't always have to take place in bed - try doing it in the shower or bath, in the kitchen, or even in the car. Experimenting with different positions, such as standing up or lying on the side, can also add a new level of excitement.

Another way to change things up is by incorporating different sensual experiences into your oral sex routine. You can try using flavored lubes or warming gels, or even experiment with different types of foods like whipped cream or chocolate sauce that can be incorporated in the oral sex experience.

Role play is another creative way to add excitement. Try out different characters or scenarios, such as doctor and patient, teacher and student, or even superhero and villain. This can add a whole new level of excitement and anticipation.

Toys can also be incorporated into oral sex sessions. For example, couples can use sex toys like vibrators that can be placed on the clitoris or on the head of the penis during oral sex. Oral beads can also be introduced to enhance the sensation and rhythm of a blowjob.

Another way to make it more exciting and creative is to play erotic games. It can be anything from strip poker to adult truth or dare games. These games can help loosen up both partners, bring them closer together, and keep things interesting.

**Avoiding Boredom in the Bedroom**

One of the biggest challenges in any long-term relationship is avoiding boredom in the bedroom. Here are some tips that can help you keep your oral sex sessions fresh and exciting:

**Communication**: Talk to your partner about what they like, what they don't like, and what they want to try. Be open and honest with each other so that you both can explore each other's sexual desires.

**Mix it up:** Try new positions, new techniques, or new locations. Don't be afraid to experiment and try new things.

**Surprise your partner**: Surprise your partner with unexpected actions or effects. For example, blindfolding them, changing the temperature of the room, or using a mask or roleplaying can be exciting and new.

**Introduce sensory play**: Incorporate things like ice cubes, hot wax, or feathers into oral sex routines for added sensation and pleasure. Sensory play can help involve more senses in the experience, making it more enjoyable and memorable.

**Take your time**: Oral sex isn't a race, and it doesn't need to be rushed. Take your time and explore every inch of your partner's body, focusing on their reactions and what they enjoy most.

**Focus on pleasure, not just orgasm**: While orgasm is often the goal of sexual activity, it's important to focus on pleasure as well. Taking pleasure in the sensations, intimacy, and connection of oral sex can make the experience much more fulfilling for both partners.

In conclusion, mixing things up and avoiding boredom in the bedroom is essential for keeping a relationship healthy and happy. By exploring new positions, incorporating toys and sensory play, and focusing on pleasure rather than just orgasm, couples can keep their oral sex sessions fresh and exciting for years to come. Remember to communicate openly with your partner, be adventurous, and most importantly, have fun. With these tips and ideas, you can spice up your sex life and enjoy more satisfying oral sex experiences together.

# Chapter 7

## Q&A with Sex Experts

In this chapter, we have invited some sex experts to provide advice and tips on oral sex and to answer some of the common questions and concerns that couples may have.

**Expert Advice and Tips on Oral Sex**

**"Communication is Key"** - Dr. Susan Simpson, a licensed clinical psychologist and sex therapist, recommends that couples prioritize communication when it comes to oral sex. She suggests that partners should talk about what feels good, what they like or don't like, and also to ask for what they want.

**"Don't Neglect the Balls"** - Samantha Jones, a sex educator, emphasizes on the importance of paying attention to the testicles during oral sex. She suggests using hands and tongue to stimulate the balls and scrotum, which can enhance the overall pleasure for both partners.

**"Vary Your Technique"** - Dr. Michael Smith, an urologist and sexual health expert, advises couples to vary their oral sex technique to avoid boredom or predictability. This can mean trying different positions, applying different pressures or speeds, or even incorporating some gentle teeth play for added sensation.

**"Take your time"** - Sex therapist and educator Eliza Paterson recommends taking your time during oral sex, as rushing can lead to an unsatisfactory experience. She suggests using slow, tantalizing movement and focusing on building anticipation before moving on to more intense stimulations.

## Common Questions and Concerns Answered

### Can oral sex increase the risk of STDs?

Yes, oral sex can transmit sexually transmitted infections such as HIV, gonorrhea, chlamydia, syphilis, and herpes. It's important to use appropriate barrier protection such as dental dams or condoms during oral sex to reduce the risk of transmission.

### I feel self-conscious about performing oral sex on my partner. What should I do?

It's not uncommon to feel self-conscious about performing oral sex, especially if it's a new experience. Dr. Susan Simpson suggests talking to your partner about your concerns, and perhaps exploring ways to build your confidence before engaging in oral sex. Remember that pleasure is a two-way street and your partner likely wants you to feel comfortable and enjoy yourself as well.

## My partner ejaculates quickly during oral sex. Is there anything we can do to prolong the experience?

Premature ejaculation during oral sex can be frustrating for both partners. Dr. Michael Smith recommends trying techniques such as edging, where the partner is brought close to orgasm multiple times before ultimately being allowed to ejaculate. Another approach is to use desensitizing sprays or creams to temporarily reduce sensitivity and prolong the experience.

## Is it normal to not orgasm from oral sex?

Yes, it's perfectly normal to not orgasm from oral sex. Everyone experiences pleasure differently, and some may find it more difficult to orgasm from oral stimulation than others. Experts suggest focusing on the sensation and pleasure rather than achieving orgasm as the main goal.

## How can I make sure my partner is comfortable and enjoying oral sex?

Communication is key in ensuring that your partner is comfortable and enjoying themselves during oral sex. Check in with them regularly, and pay attention to their verbal and nonverbal cues to gauge their level of pleasure and comfort. Make sure to be responsive to your partner's needs and preferences, and don't hesitate to ask for feedback or directions from them.

By following the expert advice and addressing common questions and concerns, couples can feel more confident and enjoy a fulfilling oral sex experience. Remember that oral sex should focus on pleasure rather than pressure or expectations, and it's important to communicate openly and prioritize your partner's enjoyment and comfort. With these tips, couples can take their sex lives to new heights of intimacy and connection.

Cheryl Bach

45

# Chapter 8

## Troubleshooting

While oral sex can be a pleasurable and satisfying sexual experience, it's not uncommon to encounter common issues that can dampen the mood. In this chapter, we will address some common issues during oral sex and provide tips for problem-solving in the moment.

**Common Issues during Oral Sex**

**Dry Mouth** - A very common issue is experiencing a dry mouth during oral sex. This can make the experience less pleasurable for both partners and lead to discomfort or pain.

**Teeth Sensitivity** - Sensitivity or pain caused by teeth during oral sex can also be a common problem for many couples.

**Difficulty Reaching Orgasm-** Some individuals may experience difficulty reaching orgasm during oral sex, which can be frustrating and affect their overall enjoyment of the experience.

## Tips for Problem-Solving in the Moment

**Address Dry Mouth** – If you are experiencing dry mouth during oral sex, try using water-based lubrication or drinking water beforehand to keep your mouth wet and comfortable. Sugary beverages should be avoided as they can lead to yeast infections. Additionally, you can switch between oral sex and manual stimulation to give your mouth a break.

**Teeth Sensitivity** - It's essential to communicate with your partner about their sensitivity to teeth during oral sex. It may be necessary to avoid contact with the teeth altogether or limit it to certain techniques like lightly brushing them against the skin. Using a flavored dental dam or condom could be helpful to prevent direct contact with the teeth.

**Difficulty Reaching Orgasm** - If one partner is struggling to reach orgasm, communicate about what works for them. Experimenting with different techniques, changing positions, or adding some foreplay could make the experience more pleasurable. Do not pressure your partner to reach orgasm and keep in mind that it's an experience to enjoy, not a goal to achieve. Don't be afraid to try something new, and remember that open communication can go a long way in improving the overall experience.

**Take Breaks** - Oral sex should be enjoyed in a comfortable and relaxed environment. If you or your partner experience

Cheryl Bach

discomfort or fatigue, take a break. A couple can use this opportunity to switch positions, experiment with different techniques, or talk dirty which could bring in a new dimension of pleasure.

**Mindset** - Maintaining a positive mindset can help avoid any distractions that could impact the experience negatively. Creating positive mental images rather than focusing on negative or nervous thoughts can enhance the mood. For instance, visualizing an intimate moment or erotic fantasies can spice things up.

**To Sum Up**

Oral sex comes with its own set of challenges, but effective communication, creativity, and patience can make the experience more enjoyable for both partners. By addressing common issues during oral sex such as dry mouth, sensitivity or pain from teeth, difficulty reaching orgasm, keeping a positive mindset, and taking breaks to switch things up, couples can create a gratifying and satisfying sexual connection. Keep an open mind about trying new methods and finding what works best for you and your partner. Improving oral sex isn't just about physical technique; it also involves emotional intimacy, trust, and mutual respect. Ultimately, couples who prioritize their partner's satisfaction, respect boundaries, and remain attentive to cues can create a thriving, healthy sexual relationship.

Cheryl Bach

# Chapter 9

## Moving Forward

Oral sex can be a fun and fantastic way to connect with your partner. However, for many couples, an unhealthy approach to sex can cause confusion, insecurity, hurt, and mistrust. In this chapter, we will discuss developing a healthy sexual lifestyle centered on consent, boundaries, and mutual respect.

**Developing a Healthy Sexual Lifestyle**

A healthy sexual lifestyle involves open communication between partners, prioritizing pleasure and satisfaction for both parties, and creating an environment that feels physically and emotionally safe. Here are some tips for developing a healthy sex life:

**Communicate**: Proper communication and dialogue about sexual needs, desires, and boundaries is essential to maintaining a healthy sex life. Speak openly and honestly with your partner, listen actively, and respect their feelings and opinions.

**Be Respectful**: Respect each other's boundaries, desires, and preferences. Always ask for consent, respect your partner's decisions and feel free to make your own.

**Prioritize Pleasure**: Sexual experiences should be mutually satisfying and enjoyable. Try out new things, share information, fantasies and ensure you are open to each other about what works and doesn't.

**Take Safety Measures**: Whether you're practicing oral sex, intercourse, or any sex act, adopting healthy practices like getting STI tests, using protection like condoms or dental dams, cleaning up surroundings (in case of stimulation during dinner), or lubricants can promote your physical safety and reduce the risk of sexually transmitted infections.

**Creating an erotic environment**: A perfect ambiance with a few touches like sensual lighting, soft music, erotic scents, and candlelight can work wonders to create a relaxing, stress-free atmosphere. Any anxiety in doing something new or different that resonates with your partner, an erotic environment will help to lower your guard and make you feel a lot more comfortable.

## Consenting, Boundaries, and Mutual Respect

Consent is the foundation of a healthy sexual lifestyle. It involves ensuring that both partners participate in any sexual activity willingly and explicitly agree on where the boundaries and limits lie. Here's some insight on how to incorporate consent into your sex life:

Cheryl Bach

**Get Explicit Consent**: Consent can only be given explicitly. This means that both parties need to communicate freely, openly, and positively about their desires and consent to any act. The absence of a "no" does not mean there is consent.

**Respect Your Partner's Boundaries**: Always respect your partner's boundaries during sexual experiences. Do not pursue acts that are uncomfortable or unwanted if you are unsure of their partner's preferences.

**Remember Your Boundaries**: Just as it's important to respect your partner's boundaries, you should be mindful of your own. Become aware of your boundaries and preferences to communicate them clearly to your partner.

**Re-evaluate Boundaries Over Time:** Your personal boundaries may change over time, so it's essential to evaluate them regularly. Approach these conversations in healthy and non-judgmental ways with your partner.

**Be Mindful of Non-Verbal Cues**: Keep an eye on your partner's non-verbal cues like body language and facial expressions. These can help in understanding whether they are comfortable or uncomfortable during the sexual experience.

**Promote Mutual Respect**: Sexual experiences should be all about mutual respect. Patients with different opinions, respecting and accepting the communication style of the partner, allowing the freedom and being responsive are some of the ways to promote mutual respect.

**Apologize and Correct Mistakes**: Recognizing when we have hurt our partners during sexual interactions is crucial to developing a culture of mutual respect. If partners feel violated or uncomfortable, it's essential to apologize, recognize the behavior and correct it in a healthy and respectful way.

In summary, incorporating consent, boundaries, and mutual respect into your oral sex life will fundamentally improve how you and your partner view your sex life. Open communication, respecting each other's preferences, valuing boundaries, and promoting mutual respect create an environment of safety, vulnerability, and trust in your sexual relationship. Building a healthy sexual lifestyle will lead to a positive sense of intimacy with your partner, heightened pleasure, and shared satisfaction that can significantly enhance your romantic relationship for long-lasting happiness.

# Conclusion

Thank you for taking the time to explore the world of oral sex with us. We hope this guide has provided you with the knowledge, skills, and inspiration to enhance your sexual experiences and bring a new level of pleasure and intimacy to your relationship.

By prioritizing communication, consent, and trust, you and your partner can create a safe and enjoyable space for exploring oral sex. By experimenting with new techniques and positions, you can discover what works for you as individuals and as a couple. And by embracing the joy and playfulness that comes with exploring one another's bodies, you can deepen your emotional connection and strengthen your bond as lovers.

Above all, remember that the most important aspect of any sexual experience is that both partners enjoy and feel comfortable throughout. Don't be afraid to share your desires and boundaries with your partner. Use the tips and techniques in this guide as a starting point, but always listen to your body and trust your instincts.

We hope this handbook has helped you embrace the joys of oral sex and opened up new possibilities for exploration and intimacy in your relationship. Remember to communicate openly and often, prioritize consent and trust, and above all, have fun!

Thank you for joining us on this journey and we wish you many pleasurable and intimate moments ahead.